Dr. Barbar for Arthritis

The Ultimate Guide on Treating and Curing Arthritis with Natural Barbara O'Neill Recommended Herbs and Foods

ISBN 978-1-300-54185-1
Theodore Jamieson
Copyright@2025

TABLE OF CONTENT

CHAPTER 1

Introduction

A Concise Look at Arthritis and Its Effects on People

Arthritis refers to a variety of conditions that impact the joints, leading to inflammation, discomfort, and rigidity. This common issue influences countless people around the globe, greatly affecting their overall well-being. The two most prevalent forms of arthritis are osteoarthritis and rheumatoid arthritis.

Osteoarthritis is a condition that affects the joints, leading to the gradual deterioration of the cartilage that serves as a cushion between the bones. It usually impacts the hands, knees, hips, and spine. This condition often comes with the passage of time, yet various elements like joint injuries, excess weight, and hereditary factors can also play a role in its emergence. Signs of osteoarthritis encompass discomfort in the joints, sensitivity, rigidity, and a decrease in flexibility. As the condition advances, it may result in the formation of bone spurs and a total depletion of cartilage, leading to heightened discomfort and reduced movement.

Rheumatoid arthritis is an autoimmune condition where the immune system erroneously targets the synovium, the lining of the joints. This results in discomfort, tenderness, and inflammation in the impacted joints. As time goes on, rheumatoid arthritis may lead to changes in joint structure and deterioration of the bones. This condition typically influences the small joints in the hands and feet, but it can also have effects on various other organs and systems throughout the body. Signs of rheumatoid arthritis encompass discomfort in the joints, inflammation, rigidity (notably upon waking), tiredness, and elevated temperature.

The effects of arthritis on individuals can be significant. The persistent discomfort and rigidity linked to the condition can hinder everyday tasks and diminish overall physical capability. Individuals experiencing arthritis often struggle with everyday activities like walking, ascending stairs, or even holding onto items. This may result in a diminished quality of life, emotional turmoil, and feelings of loneliness. Furthermore, the financial impact of arthritis is significant, encompassing expenses for medical care, prescriptions, and decreased productivity. Introduction to Dr. Barbara O'Neill and Her Approach to Holistic Healing

Dr. Barbara O'Neill is a respected expert in natural health and education, committed to advocating for holistic methods to enhance well-being and vitality. With a background in nutrition and holistic approaches, Dr. O'Neill emphasizes the importance of addressing the root causes of health issues rather than just managing symptoms. Her approach to treating arthritis involves a combination of dietary changes, lifestyle modifications, and the use of holistic solutions to reduce inflammation, alleviate pain, and support overall joint health.

Dr. O'Neill's philosophy emphasizes the idea that the body possesses a natural capacity for self-healing when provided with the appropriate support and surroundings. She champions the use of wholesome foods and botanical solutions to enhance the body's healing abilities and alleviate inflammation. Dr. O'Neill notes that various long-term health issues, such as arthritis, can be worsened by unhealthy eating and lifestyle practices. By embracing beneficial adjustments in these areas, individuals can enhance their overall well-being and alleviate the intensity of their arthritis symptoms.

One of the key aspects of Dr. O'Neill's approach is the incorporation of soothing herbs and nourishing foods. She suggests adding herbs like ginger, turmeric, boswellia, and devil's claw to your meals. These herbs are known for their remarkable ability to alleviate joint pain and inflammation effectively. For instance, turmeric has curcumin, a substance recognized for its capacity to block inflammatory pathways within the body. In a similar vein, ginger has a long history of being utilized for its soothing and pain-relieving properties.

Alongside herbal options, Dr. O'Neill highlights the significance of incorporating a diet abundant in alkaline and anti-inflammatory foods. Foods that are rich in alkalinity, like dark green leafy vegetables, fruits, and specific grains, can assist in balancing the body's pH levels and minimizing inflammation. Foods that help reduce inflammation, including berries, fatty fish, nuts, seeds, and olive oil, offer vital nutrients that promote joint health and lessen oxidative stress. Dr. O'Neill emphasizes the significance of staying hydrated, as consuming enough water is essential for keeping joints lubricated and supporting overall well-being.

Dr. O'Neill's approach emphasizes holistic lifestyle changes that may alleviate arthritis symptoms and enhance overall wellness. Consistent movement is a fundamental part of her suggestions, as engaging in physical activity promotes joint flexibility, fortifies muscles, and alleviates discomfort. She inspires people to participate in gentle activities like swimming, walking, and yoga. Furthermore, practices like meditation, yoga, and deep breathing exercises are suggested to assist in managing the emotional and psychological challenges associated with living with arthritis.

Another important aspect of Dr. O'Neill's approach is the use of holistic treatments and therapies. For example, she promotes the use of hydrotherapy, which incorporates hot and cold applications to alleviate inflammation and ease discomfort. Ginger poultices, created by blending ginger with water and applying them to the affected joints, are suggested for their soothing and pain-relieving properties. Breathing exercises, which enhance oxygen flow to the cells, are an essential component of her comprehensive approach to wellness.

Throughout her career, Dr. Barbara O'Neill has empowered countless individuals to alleviate their arthritis symptoms and enhance their quality of life using gentle and holistic approaches. Her approach focuses on holistic principles, highlighting the significance of addressing the entire individual—mind, body, and spirit. By focusing on the root causes of arthritis and enhancing the body's innate healing abilities, Dr. O'Neill's suggestions provide a hopeful option for those looking for a more organic and comprehensive way to manage their condition, as opposed to traditional treatments.

CHAPTER 2

Understanding Arthritis

Definition and Types of Arthritis

Arthritis is a term used to describe over 100 different conditions that cause pain, swelling, and stiffness in the joints. It is a leading cause of disability, affecting millions of people worldwide. The word arthritis itself is derived from the Greek words arthro (joint) and itis (inflammation), which accurately reflects the primary characteristic of these conditions: joint inflammation.

The most common types of arthritis include:

Osteoarthritis (OA): This is the most prevalent form of arthritis, often referred to as wear and tear arthritis. It occurs when the cartilage that cushions the ends of bones in the joints gradually deteriorates. As the cartilage wears away, bones can rub against each other, causing pain, swelling, and reduced joint mobility. OA typically affects weight-bearing joints such as the knees, hips, and spine, as well as the hands.

Rheumatoid Arthritis (RA): RA is an autoimmune disease in which the body's immune system mistakenly attacks the synovium—the lining of the membranes that surround the joints. This leads to inflammation, pain, and swelling. Over time, RA can cause joint deformity and erosion of the bones. RA often affects the small joints of the hands and feet but can also impact other organs and systems in the body.

Psoriatic Arthritis (PsA): This type of arthritis occurs in some individuals with psoriasis, a skin condition characterized by red, scaly patches. PsA can cause joint pain, stiffness, and swelling, and it often affects the fingers and toes. It can also lead to changes in the nails and cause inflammation in other parts of the body, such as the eyes.

Ankylosing Spondylitis (AS): AS is a type of inflammatory arthritis that primarily affects the spine. It causes inflammation of the vertebrae, leading to chronic pain and stiffness. In severe cases, the inflammation can cause the vertebrae to fuse, resulting in a loss of flexibility and a hunched posture.

Gout: Gout is a form of arthritis caused by the accumulation of uric acid crystals in the joints. It often affects the big toe but can also occur in other joints such as the ankles, knees, and wrists. Gout attacks are characterized by sudden, severe pain, redness, and swelling.

Common Symptoms and Causes

The symptoms of arthritis can vary depending on the type and severity of the condition, but common symptoms include:

Joint Pain: Pain is the most prominent symptom of arthritis. It can range from mild to severe and may be constant or intermittent.

Swelling: Inflammation in the joints can cause swelling and tenderness.

Stiffness: Joint stiffness is especially common in the morning or after periods of inactivity.

Reduced Range of Motion: Arthritis can limit the flexibility and movement of the affected joints.

Redness and Warmth: In some types of arthritis, the affected joints may appear red and feel warm to the touch.

Fatigue: Chronic pain and inflammation can lead to feelings of fatigue and reduced energy levels.

Joint Deformity: In severe cases, arthritis can cause visible changes in the shape of the joints.

The causes of arthritis can be complex and multifactorial. Some common causes and risk factors include:

Age: The risk of developing arthritis increases with age, particularly for osteoarthritis.

Genetics: A family history of arthritis can increase the likelihood of developing the condition.

Gender: Some types of arthritis, such as rheumatoid arthritis and lupus, are more common in women, while gout is more prevalent in men.

Injury: Joint injuries or repetitive stress on the joints can increase the risk of developing arthritis later in life.

Obesity: Excess weight puts additional stress on weight-bearing joints, increasing the risk of osteoarthritis.

Infections: Certain bacterial and viral infections can trigger arthritis or make it worse.

Autoimmune Disorders: In conditions like rheumatoid arthritis, the immune system attacks the body's own tissues, leading to joint inflammation.

Metabolic Abnormalities: Conditions such as gout are caused by metabolic issues that lead to the accumulation of uric acid crystals in the joints.

The Role of Inflammation in Arthritis

Inflammation is a natural immune response to injury or infection, characterized by redness, swelling, warmth, and pain. While acute inflammation is a protective mechanism that helps the body heal, chronic inflammation can have detrimental effects on health and is a key factor in many types of arthritis.

In arthritis, inflammation primarily affects the joints, leading to pain, swelling, and stiffness. The process of inflammation involves the release of inflammatory mediators, such as cytokines and chemokines, which attract immune cells to the site of injury or infection. These immune cells produce additional inflammatory substances, perpetuating the cycle of inflammation.

In osteoarthritis (OA), inflammation is a result of the breakdown of cartilage and the body's attempt to repair the damaged joint. The wear and tear on the cartilage cause the release of pro-inflammatory mediators, which contribute to the degradation of the joint. Chronic low-grade inflammation is a hallmark of OA and plays a significant role in the progression of the disease.

In rheumatoid arthritis (RA), the inflammation is driven by an autoimmune response. The immune system attacks the synovium, causing it to become inflamed and thickened. This leads to the production of excess synovial fluid, swelling, and pain. The ongoing inflammation can damage the cartilage and bone within the joint, leading to deformity and loss of function. In RA, the inflammation is systemic, meaning it can also affect other organs and systems in the body.

Psoriatic arthritis (PsA) and ankylosing spondylitis (AS) are also characterized by chronic inflammation. In PsA, the inflammation affects both the skin and joints, leading to joint pain and skin lesions. In AS, the inflammation primarily targets the spine, causing pain and stiffness.

Gout is an example of arthritis where inflammation is triggered by the presence of uric acid crystals in the joints. These crystals are perceived as foreign by the immune system, leading to a robust inflammatory response. The sudden and severe inflammation results in intense pain and swelling.

The role of inflammation in arthritis underscores the importance of managing it to alleviate symptoms and slow disease progression. Treatment approaches often focus on reducing inflammation through medications, dietary changes, and lifestyle modifications. Anti-inflammatory drugs, such as nonsteroidal anti-inflammatory drugs (NSAIDs) and corticosteroids, are commonly used to manage arthritis symptoms. Additionally, natural anti-inflammatory remedies, such as ginger, turmeric, and omega-3 fatty acids, can be beneficial in reducing inflammation.

CHAPTER 3

Recommended Herbs for Arthritis

Ginger: A Natural Anti-Inflammatory Agent

Ginger, a popular spice and healing herb, has been revered for its powerful ability to reduce inflammation. The compounds found in ginger, particularly gingerols and shogaols, are recognized for their ability to reduce inflammation and provide antioxidant benefits, which may assist in easing the symptoms of arthritis.

Ginger functions by reducing the creation of certain substances that contribute to inflammation, including specific enzymes and cytokines that are vital to the body's inflammatory processes. By lowering the levels of these inflammatory substances, ginger can assist in alleviating joint pain and swelling linked to arthritis.

Alongside its anti-inflammatory benefits, ginger also has pain-relieving qualities, making it a powerful option for alleviating discomfort. Research indicates that ginger may alleviate discomfort and enhance mobility in those suffering from osteoarthritis and rheumatoid arthritis.

Ginger can be enjoyed in multiple ways, such as fresh ginger root, ginger tea, ginger supplements, and ginger extract.
Turmeric: The Power of Curcumin and Its Advantages

Turmeric is a remarkable herb known for its anti-inflammatory properties, utilized for centuries in age-old healing practices. The main active ingredient in turmeric, curcumin, is known for its various health advantages, such as its capacity to lessen inflammation and ease arthritis symptoms.

Curcumin functions by blocking the action of enzymes and cytokines that promote inflammation, including COX-2, TNF-alpha, and interleukins. It also inhibits the activation of nuclear factor-kappa B (NF-kB), an important regulator of the body's inflammatory response. By influencing these pathways, curcumin may assist in alleviating joint inflammation, discomfort, and rigidity.

Studies indicate that curcumin may provide similar benefits to nonsteroidal anti-inflammatory drugs (NSAIDs) for alleviating arthritis symptoms, while avoiding the unwanted side effects. Moreover, curcumin offers protective benefits for the joints by combating oxidative stress and damage through its antioxidant qualities.

Turmeric can be included in your meals in many delightful ways, like mixing it into curries, soups, and smoothies, or opting for turmeric supplements. It's essential to recognize that curcumin has limited absorption, which means the body doesn't readily take it in. For better absorption, it's advisable to pair turmeric with black pepper, as the piperine in black pepper boosts the bioavailability of curcumin.

Boswellia: Alleviating Joint Discomfort

Boswellia, often referred to as Indian frankincense, is a resin sourced from the Boswellia serrata tree. It has been utilized in age-old practices for its soothing and pain-relieving qualities. The compounds found in boswellia, referred to as boswellic acids, have demonstrated the ability to reduce the production of pro-inflammatory enzymes and cytokines, including 5-lipoxygenase (5-LOX) and leukotrienes.

By addressing these inflammatory mediators, boswellic acids may assist in alleviating joint inflammation and discomfort for those experiencing arthritis. Studies indicate that boswellia may enhance symptoms associated with osteoarthritis and rheumatoid arthritis, such as discomfort, rigidity, and overall physical performance.

Boswellia comes in a range of options, such as capsules, tablets, and topical creams. It can be used as a supplement or applied directly to the affected joints for targeted comfort. Before incorporating boswellia into your routine, it's essential to seek guidance from a healthcare professional, particularly if you are on other medications or have existing health issues.

Devil's Claw: Soothing Discomfort and Reducing Inflammation

Devil's claw is a plant from southern Africa, recognized for its unique hooked fruit and healing qualities. The active compounds in devil's claw, known as harpagosides, have demonstrated anti-inflammatory and analgesic properties, which contributes to its popularity for alleviating arthritis symptoms.

Harpagosides function by reducing the creation of substances that promote inflammation, including COX-2 and nitric oxide synthase. By minimizing inflammation, devil's claw can assist in easing joint discomfort, swelling, and rigidity linked to arthritis. Moreover, devil's claw has demonstrated the ability to enhance physical function and mobility in those dealing with osteoarthritis and rheumatoid arthritis.

Devil's claw comes in a variety of forms, such as capsules, tablets, and extracts. It can be utilized as a supplement or applied directly for targeted comfort. Before using devil's claw, it's essential to seek advice from a healthcare professional, particularly if you are on other medications or have existing health issues.

Additional Helpful Botanicals

Alongside ginger, turmeric, boswellia, and devil's claw, there are various other herbs that exhibit soothing and pain-relieving qualities, offering support for those dealing with arthritis:

Willow bark is known for its salicin content, which the body transforms into salicylic acid. Salicylic acid shares properties with aspirin, offering soothing and pain-relieving benefits. Willow bark may assist in alleviating joint discomfort and swelling for those experiencing arthritis.

Cat's Claw: This vine, originating from the Amazon rainforest, is celebrated for its ability to support the immune system and reduce inflammation. This formulation features elements that block the creation of pro-inflammatory substances, potentially alleviating discomfort and swelling in those experiencing rheumatoid arthritis.

Eucalyptus leaves are rich in tannins and flavonoids, which are known for their soothing and pain-relieving properties. Eucalyptus oil can be applied directly to the skin to help ease joint discomfort and swelling related to arthritis.

Green tea is rich in polyphenols, including epigallocatechin gallate (EGCG), known for its strong anti-inflammatory and antioxidant benefits. Incorporating green tea into your daily routine may aid in alleviating inflammation and safeguarding the joints against oxidative stress.

Nettle: This herb has a long history of use for its ability to reduce inflammation. This product features elements that help to limit the creation of substances that promote inflammation, potentially easing discomfort and swelling in those experiencing arthritis.

Capsaicin is a compound derived from chili peppers known for its soothing effects on discomfort. When used on the skin, capsaicin may alleviate joint discomfort by lowering the amounts of substance P, a neurotransmitter that plays a role in signaling pain.

Feverfew is a plant recognized for its soothing properties and ability to alleviate discomfort. This product features elements that can help lessen the creation of substances that promote inflammation, potentially easing discomfort and swelling in those experiencing arthritis.

These herbs can be utilized on their own or together to assist in alleviating arthritis symptoms. As with any holistic approach, it is important to consult with a healthcare professional before using these herbs, especially if you are taking other medications or have underlying health conditions.

CHAPTER 4

Foods to Eat and Avoid for Arthritis

Foods to Include in Your Diet
Foods that promote a balanced pH

1. Lemons: While lemons are commonly perceived as acidic because of their tart flavor, they surprisingly promote an alkalizing effect on the body after digestion. Lemons are packed with vitamin C, antioxidants, and bioflavonoids that bolster immune health and help alleviate inflammation. Adding lemons to your meals can assist in balancing the body's pH levels and enhance overall well-being. Incorporating lemon juice into your water, salads, and meals can elevate the taste while providing the advantages of this refreshing fruit.

2. Dark Green Leafy Vegetables: Varieties like spinach, kale, Swiss chard, and collard greens are rich in alkalinity and loaded with vital nutrients. These vegetables are abundant in essential vitamins A, C, and K, along with vital minerals such as calcium, magnesium, and potassium. These substances are rich in beneficial compounds that aid in

minimizing inflammation and promoting the well-being of joints. Incorporating a range of dark green leafy vegetables into your meals can support a balanced pH level and offer a wealth of health advantages.

3. Fruits: Numerous fruits possess alkalizing qualities and are abundant in vitamins, minerals, and antioxidants. Among the fruits that promote alkalinity, you'll find apples, pears, berries, melons, and citrus varieties. These fruits may aid in alleviating inflammation, enhancing immune function, and promoting general well-being. Incorporating a diverse selection of fruits into your diet is essential for obtaining a broad spectrum of nutrients and antioxidants.

4. Millet: This grain is wonderfully alkaline and free from gluten, packed with fiber, protein, and vital minerals. It is gentle on the stomach and may assist in harmonizing the body's pH levels. Millet serves as a wonderful alternative to rice or other grains in a variety of dishes, enhancing the versatility of your meals.

5. Quinoa: This remarkable grain is not only alkaline but also packed with protein, fiber, and essential amino acids. It provides a wealth of vitamins and

minerals, such as magnesium, iron, and potassium. The soothing qualities of quinoa make it a wonderful option for those dealing with arthritis. This ingredient is perfect for enhancing salads, enriching soups, and serving as a delightful side to accompany numerous dishes.

6. Buckwheat: Contrary to what its name suggests, buckwheat is not associated with wheat and is free from gluten. This grain boasts an alkaline nature and is rich in protein, fiber, and vital nutrients. Buckwheat boasts a wealth of antioxidants, especially rutin, known for its soothing anti-inflammatory effects. This ingredient is versatile and can be incorporated into pancakes, porridge, or used as a delightful base for salads.

7. Spelt: This ancient grain offers a gentler option for digestion compared to contemporary wheat. This substance boasts alkalizing qualities and is abundant in protein, fiber, vitamins, and minerals. Spelt serves as a wonderful option in baking, offering a delightful alternative to wheat in numerous recipes, and it can also be enjoyed as a wholesome grain in salads and side dishes.

8. Kamut: This ancient grain boasts alkalizing properties. It boasts a greater amount of protein and vital nutrients compared to contemporary wheat and is recognized for its soothing properties. Kamut is a wonderful addition to salads, soups, and as a side dish, promoting overall wellness and helping to alleviate inflammation.

9. Almonds and Brazil Nuts: These nuts are known for their alkaline properties and are packed with healthy fats, protein, fiber, vitamins, and minerals. Almonds provide a wealth of vitamin E and magnesium, and Brazil nuts stand out as a notable source of selenium, known for its strong antioxidant properties. Incorporating these nuts into your meals can promote a reduction in inflammation, enhance joint wellness, and help sustain a balanced alkaline pH level.
Foods That Help Reduce Inflammation

1. Berries: Blueberries, strawberries, raspberries, and blackberries are packed with antioxidants, vitamins, and fiber. These substances include anthocyanins and quercetin, known for their strong ability to reduce inflammation. Incorporating a mix of berries into your diet can aid in lowering inflammation, safeguarding joint health, and enhancing overall wellness. Berries can be savored

in their fresh form, enjoyed frozen, or incorporated into smoothies, salads, and delightful desserts.

2. Fatty Fish: Varieties like salmon, mackerel, sardines, and trout are wonderful sources of omega-3 fatty acids. Omega-3s possess remarkable qualities that may alleviate discomfort and rigidity in those experiencing arthritis. They contribute positively to cardiovascular wellness and enhance general vitality. Incorporating fatty fish into your meals a couple of times each week can offer remarkable health advantages. If you don't eat fish, you might want to explore a premium omega-3 supplement sourced from algae.

3. Nuts: Walnuts, almonds, and pistachios are packed with beneficial fats, protein, fiber, vitamins, and minerals. Walnuts stand out for their richness in omega-3 fatty acids, known for their soothing properties against inflammation. Incorporating a diverse selection of nuts into your meals can aid in minimizing inflammation, promote joint wellness, and deliver vital nutrients for your overall health. Nuts offer a delightful option for snacking, can enhance the flavor of salads, and serve as a versatile ingredient in both cooking and baking.

4. Seeds: Chia seeds, flaxseeds, and hemp seeds are abundant in omega-3 fatty acids, fiber, and vital nutrients. Chia seeds and flaxseeds are rich in alpha-linolenic acid (ALA), a form of omega-3 fatty acid known for its soothing effects on inflammation. Adding seeds to your meals can promote a decrease in inflammation and enhance the well-being of your joints. These can be incorporated into smoothies, yogurt, oatmeal, and baked treats.

5. Olive Oil: A staple in the Mediterranean diet, olive oil is celebrated for its soothing qualities that help reduce inflammation. It features oleocanthal, a substance that exhibits effects akin to those of nonsteroidal anti-inflammatory medications. Extra virgin olive oil boasts a wealth of monounsaturated fats and antioxidants, promoting heart health and enhancing overall wellness. Incorporating olive oil as your main cooking oil and in salad dressings can offer notable health advantages and assist in alleviating inflammation.

Staying hydrated: The significance of consuming enough water

Staying well-hydrated is crucial for promoting overall well-being and aiding in the proper functioning of your joints. Water is an essential component of the body's tissues and plays a vital role in numerous bodily functions, such as digestion, circulation, temperature control, and the removal of waste. For those dealing with arthritis, maintaining proper hydration is crucial for a variety of reasons:

1. Joint Lubrication: Staying hydrated aids in keeping the joints well-lubricated by preserving the thickness of synovial fluid, which serves as a protective cushion and minimizes friction between cartilage surfaces. Staying well-hydrated helps maintain the right balance of synovial fluid, which can alleviate discomfort and tightness in the joints.

2. Cartilage Health: The connective tissue that cushions the ends of bones in the joints is mainly made up of water. Staying well-hydrated supports the health and flexibility of cartilage, minimizing the chances of deterioration. When the body lacks sufficient hydration, it can result in the deterioration of cartilage, which heightens the chances of developing osteoarthritis.

3. Soothing Inflammation: Staying well-hydrated can assist in calming inflammation by helping to eliminate toxins and waste from the body. Not staying properly hydrated can cause

inflammatory substances to build up, making arthritis symptoms worse. Staying well-hydrated aids in the body's inherent cleansing functions and lessens the strain on the kidneys and liver.

4. Pain Management: Staying well-hydrated may ease discomfort linked to arthritis. Not staying properly hydrated can result in muscle cramps and heightened sensitivity to discomfort. Keeping your body well-hydrated supports muscle performance and can lessen the feeling of discomfort.

5. Overall Wellness: Staying hydrated is crucial for maintaining good health and vitality. It enhances digestive health, boosts nutrient uptake, elevates energy levels, and sharpens cognitive abilities. Staying well-hydrated contributes to radiant skin and supports a smooth metabolic process.

To maintain proper hydration, it's essential to consume enough water during the day. The quantity of water required can differ depending on various factors like age, weight, activity level, and climate. It's often suggested to consume around eight 8-ounce glasses of water daily, though personal requirements can differ. Moreover, incorporating foods that are rich in moisture, like juicy fruits and crisp vegetables (for instance, cucumbers, watermelon, oranges, and celery), can enhance your overall hydration levels.

Foods to Avoid
Foods with high acidity

1. Sugar: This sweet substance is quite acidic and may lead to increased inflammation within the body. Eating large quantities of sugar can result in a rise in pro-inflammatory cytokines and oxidative stress levels. This may worsen symptoms associated with arthritis, such as discomfort and rigidity. Moreover, consuming sugar can contribute to weight gain, which adds additional strain on the joints. It is essential to reduce the consumption of sweet treats and drinks, including candies, pastries, sodas, and sugary cereals. Instead, choose wholesome sweeteners such as honey or maple syrup, but use them sparingly.

2. Meat: Some varieties of meat, especially red and processed options, may contribute to an acidic environment in the body. These substances are rich in saturated fats and advanced glycation end products (AGEs), which may contribute to inflammation. Cutting back on red meat, including beef, lamb, and pork, may aid in alleviating arthritis

symptoms. Opt for lean proteins such as poultry, fish, and plant-based options like beans, lentils, and tofu.
Incorporating more meals that are derived from plants into your diet can be quite advantageous.

3. Hybridized Wheat: This type of wheat, prevalent in contemporary products, has undergone modifications to enhance its yield and pest resistance. This variety of wheat may cause inflammation in certain people, resulting in digestive discomfort and joint pain. Moreover, products made from wheat frequently have gluten, which may provoke inflammation in those who are sensitive to gluten or have celiac disease. To alleviate inflammation, think about swapping out hybridized wheat for ancient grains such as spelt, kamut, quinoa, and buckwheat. These options are gentler on the body and can offer vital nutrients.

4. Aged Cheese: Cheeses that have been aged, like cheddar, parmesan, and blue cheese, contain higher levels of saturated fats and histamines, potentially contributing to inflammation. Histamines are substances that may provoke allergic responses and worsen arthritis symptoms. Reducing the intake of aged cheeses may assist in alleviating inflammation and joint discomfort.

Instead, choose fresh cheeses such as ricotta or cottage cheese, but enjoy them in moderation. Furthermore, think about adding cheese substitutes derived from nuts or seeds to your diet.

5. Caffeine: This substance, present in coffee, tea, and certain energy drinks, can bring about a mix of benefits and drawbacks for those dealing with arthritis. While moderate caffeine consumption may offer some benefits, too much can result in heightened inflammation and discomfort in the joints. Consuming caffeine may disrupt sleep, an essential factor in alleviating arthritis symptoms. To lessen the effects of caffeine, try to keep your consumption to just one or two cups of coffee or tea each day, and steer clear of caffeine in the late afternoon or evening. Choose soothing herbal infusions and other refreshing drinks to maintain hydration.

6. Alcohol: Consuming alcohol may lead to increased inflammation and worsen symptoms associated with arthritis. It may hinder the body's capacity to take in vital nutrients and upset the harmony of gut bacteria, resulting in heightened inflammation. Moreover, consuming alcohol can hinder liver performance, an essential component for cleansing the body and alleviating swelling. To alleviate

arthritis symptoms, it is essential to reduce or completely eliminate alcohol intake. If you decide to indulge, consider doing so mindfully and select beverages with lower alcohol content, such as light beer or wine.

7. Tobacco: The use of tobacco, whether through smoking or chewing, can lead to increased inflammation and may exacerbate symptoms of arthritis. Smoking may hinder circulation to the joints, affecting the supply of oxygen and nutrients essential for their repair. It may also elevate oxidative stress and encourage the release of pro-inflammatory cytokines. Stopping tobacco use is a powerful method to decrease inflammation and enhance overall well-being. Consider reaching out to healthcare experts, community support networks, and programs designed to assist you in your journey to quit.

Artificial Foods and Sugar Additives

1. Packaged Foods: Packaged foods frequently contain unhealthy fats, refined sugars, and synthetic additives, all of which may lead to increased inflammation. These foods often lack vital nutrients and fiber, which can negatively impact overall well-being. Commonly found in our diets are quick-

service meals, convenience snacks, pre-prepared dishes, and sweetened breakfast options. Incorporating these foods into your diet frequently may result in weight gain, heightened inflammation, and a deterioration of arthritis symptoms. To enhance joint health and alleviate inflammation, it is essential to cut back on processed foods and prioritize whole, unprocessed options.

2. Refined Sugars: Refined sugars, including white sugar and high-fructose corn syrup, are prevalent in numerous processed foods and sweetened drinks. These sugars can elevate blood sugar levels and encourage the creation of pro-inflammatory cytokines. Excessive intake of refined sugars can lead to a higher likelihood of obesity, type 2 diabetes, and heart disease, all of which may worsen arthritis symptoms. Paying close attention to food labels is essential, and steering clear of items that contain added sugars is a wise choice. Choose wholesome sources of sweetness, like fruits, honey, and maple syrup, while keeping moderation in mind.

3. Trans Fats: These fats, often referred to as partially hydrogenated oils, are frequently present in processed foods, baked goods, and fried items. These fats can lead to inflammation and may

elevate the risk of long-term health issues, such as heart disease and arthritis. Trans fats can elevate bad cholesterol (LDL) while decreasing good cholesterol (HDL), which may lead to inflammation and discomfort in the joints. For alleviating inflammation and enhancing joint wellness, steer clear of trans fats and opt for more wholesome fats like olive oil, avocado, and nuts.

4. Refined Grains: Refined grains, including white flour, white rice, and white bread, have lost their bran and germ, which are vital sources of nutrients and fiber. These grains can cause quick increases in blood sugar levels, which may contribute to heightened inflammation. Regularly consuming refined grains may lead to weight gain and worsen arthritis symptoms. For better joint health, consider swapping out refined grains for wholesome options such as quinoa, brown rice, oats, and whole wheat products. Whole grains offer a wealth of nutrients, fiber, and soothing properties that can help reduce inflammation.

5. Synthetic Additives: Numerous processed foods are loaded with synthetic additives, including preservatives, flavor enhancers, and colorings, which may lead to

inflammation and adversely affect overall well-being. It's wise to steer clear of certain additives like monosodium glutamate (MSG), artificial sweeteners such as aspartame and saccharin, as well as food colorings like Red 40 and Yellow 5. These additives may lead to allergic reactions, digestive problems, and worsen arthritis symptoms. To minimize contact with synthetic substances, opt for whole, unrefined foods and pay close attention to food labels.

6. Sodium: An excessive amount of sodium is often found in processed foods and may lead to fluid retention and elevated blood pressure. Too much sodium can contribute to heightened inflammation and discomfort in the joints. To alleviate arthritis symptoms and enhance overall well-being, it is essential to reduce sodium consumption. Steer clear of salty snacks, processed meats, canned soups, and other foods that are high in sodium. Instead, enhance your meals with the goodness of herbs, spices, and wholesome flavorings like lemon juice and garlic.

7. Fast Food: Fast food tends to be loaded with unhealthy fats, refined sugars, and sodium, contributing to inflammation and negatively impacting overall well-being. Frequent intake of

fast food may contribute to weight increase, heightened inflammation, and a deterioration of arthritis symptoms. To enhance joint health and alleviate inflammation, it's essential to cut back on fast food and choose nourishing, homemade meals crafted from whole, unprocessed ingredients.

CHAPTER 5

Natural Remedies and Therapies

Water Therapy: Warm and Cool Treatments

The therapeutic application of water has been embraced for centuries to ease discomfort, diminish swelling, and enhance overall health. One of the most effective techniques for managing arthritis symptoms is the application of hot and cold treatments. These approaches can assist in alleviating joint discomfort, boosting blood flow, and increasing flexibility.

Warm Treatments:

Warm baths, hot packs, and heating pads can be beneficial for relaxing muscles, enhancing blood circulation, and alleviating joint stiffness. The warmth expands blood vessels, enhancing blood flow and providing vital nutrients and oxygen to the impacted regions. This may alleviate discomfort and encourage recovery.

Soothing Baths: Immersing yourself in a warm bath can ease discomfort from arthritis and help alleviate stiffness. Incorporating Epsom salts into your bath can elevate the experience, as the magnesium present in the salts may aid in alleviating inflammation and soothing muscles.

Warm Compresses: Using warm compresses or heating pads on the affected joints can provide relief from discomfort and tightness. Using a barrier, like a towel, is crucial to protect against burns and to limit extended exposure to heat.

Steam rooms and saunas create a warm atmosphere that promotes muscle relaxation, alleviates joint stiffness, and enhances blood flow. Enjoying a steam room or sauna can provide relief for those dealing with arthritis.

Chilly Treatments:

Applying cold, like ice packs and compresses, can effectively ease inflammation, dull discomfort, and narrow blood vessels. This can be especially beneficial during sudden episodes when joints experience swelling and discomfort.

Cold Compresses: Using cold compresses on the affected joints can assist in minimizing swelling and numbing the area, offering relief from discomfort. Using a protective layer, like a cloth, is crucial to avoid frostbite, and it's best to limit the application to 15-20 minutes at a time.

Chilled Cloths: Chilled cloths, created by soaking a fabric in cool water and placing it on the sore joints, can offer comparable advantages to ice packs. This approach can provide a gentler experience for those who find extreme cold uncomfortable.

Contrast Hydrotherapy:

Contrast hydrotherapy consists of switching between hot and cold treatments, which may enhance circulation, alleviate discomfort, and support the healing process. This approach can be especially beneficial for alleviating the discomfort associated with arthritis.

Procedure: Start with a warm compress for 3-5 minutes, then switch to a cool compress for 1-2 minutes. Complete this process 3-5 times, concluding with a cold treatment. This approach can enhance circulation, alleviate swelling, and offer comfort from discomfort.

Ginger Poultices: How to Use and Their Advantages

Ginger poultices are a time-honored solution that utilizes the soothing and pain-relieving qualities of ginger to ease joint discomfort and swelling. A paste of ginger applied to the affected area can alleviate discomfort, enhance blood flow, and support the healing process.

Advantages of Ginger Compresses:

Ginger is rich in compounds known as gingerols and shogaols, which are recognized for their strong ability to reduce inflammation. These compounds may assist in lowering the creation of pro-inflammatory cytokines and enzymes, providing relief from joint pain and swelling.

Ginger possesses inherent properties that may alleviate pain and discomfort in the affected joints.

Circulation: Ginger enhances blood flow to the affected area, providing vital nutrients and oxygen to support the healing process.

Steps for Creating and Using a Ginger Poultice:

Ingredients:

Raw ginger root

Pure and refreshing, this essential element nourishes and revitalizes the body.

Fabric or mesh

How to Prepare:

Finely chop or grate the fresh ginger root.

Combine the grated ginger with sufficient water in a pot to ensure it's fully submerged.

Gently heat the ginger on low for 10-15 minutes to allow its beneficial properties to infuse.

Take the ginger off the heat and let it cool for a bit.

Usage:

Evenly apply the ginger paste onto a cloth or gauze.

Gently place the ginger poultice on the troubled joint, ensuring it stays in position with a soft cloth or bandage.

Keep the poultice in place for 20-30 minutes, letting the ginger seep into the skin to offer soothing comfort.

Once you take off the poultice, wash the area with warm water and softly dab it dry.

Ginger poultices may be used once or twice daily, based on how intense the symptoms are. Consistent application may aid in minimizing swelling, easing discomfort, and enhancing mobility in the joints.

Breathing Techniques: Enhancing Oxygen Delivery to Cells

Breathing exercises offer a straightforward and powerful method to boost oxygen delivery to the cells, alleviate stress, and promote a sense of overall wellness. Effective breathing methods can enhance oxygen absorption, boost circulation, and aid the body's innate recovery mechanisms. For those dealing with arthritis, adding breathing exercises to their daily routine can assist in alleviating pain, minimizing inflammation, and fostering a sense of calm.

Advantages of Breathing Techniques:

Enhanced Oxygen Flow: Utilizing effective breathing methods can boost the oxygen supply to the cells, aiding in energy generation and overall cellular activity.

Enhanced Blood Flow: Engaging in deep breathing can boost circulation, ensuring that vital nutrients and oxygen reach the joints, which aids in the healing process.

Stress Relief: Engaging in breathing exercises can stimulate the parasympathetic nervous system, fostering a sense of calm and alleviating tension. Managing stress is essential for overall well-being, as it can worsen arthritis symptoms.

Pain Management: Deep breathing can alleviate the sensation of discomfort by encouraging relaxation and triggering the release of endorphins, which are the body's own pain-relieving substances.

Varieties of Breathing Techniques:

Deep Breathing Techniques:

Diaphragmatic breathing, often referred to as abdominal or belly breathing, focuses on taking deep breaths into the diaphragm instead of shallow breaths into the chest. This method can enhance oxygen absorption and encourage a sense of calm.

Ways to Engage:

Find a cozy spot to either sit or lie down.

Gently rest one hand on your chest and the other on your abdomen.

Breathe in slowly through your nose, letting your belly expand as you take in the fresh air. Keep your chest calm and steady.

Breathe out gently through your mouth, letting your belly relax as you let the air go.

Engage in this practice for 5-10 minutes, concentrating on slow, even breaths.

Breathing with pursed lips:

Pursed-lip breathing is a method that entails taking a breath in through the nose and gently releasing it through pursed lips. This approach can enhance oxygen flow, alleviate breathlessness, and encourage a sense of calm.

Ways to Engage:

Find a cozy spot to either sit or lie down.

Breathe in slowly through your nose for a count of two.

Shape your lips as if preparing to produce a gentle sound.

Breathe out softly and calmly through your pursed lips for a count of four.

Engage in this practice for 5-10 minutes, emphasizing gentle, deliberate breathing.

Box Breathing Technique:

Box breathing, often referred to as square breathing, is a method that consists of inhaling, pausing, exhaling, and pausing once more in a rhythmic sequence. This approach can enhance concentration, alleviate tension, and encourage a sense of calm.

Ways to Engage:

Find a cozy spot where you can relax, ensuring your back is aligned and your feet rest gently on the floor.

Breathe in slowly through your nose for a count of four.

Take a deep breath and pause for a count of four.

Breathe out softly and calmly through your mouth for a count of four.

Take a deep breath and hold it for a count of four.

Engage in this practice for 5-10 minutes, ensuring you keep a consistent rhythm throughout.

Breathing Through Alternate Nostrils:

Alternate nostril breathing is a practice that entails inhaling and exhaling through one nostril at a time, while gently closing the other nostril with a finger. This approach can assist in harmonizing the nervous system, alleviating stress, and encouraging a sense of calm.

Ways to Engage:

Find a cozy spot where you can relax, ensuring your spine is aligned and upright.

Gently press your right thumb against your right nostril.

Take a slow, deep breath in through your left nostril for a count of four.

Gently press your right ring finger against your left nostril.

Take a deep breath and hold it for a count of four.

Breathe out gently through your right nostril, counting to four as you do so.

Take a slow, deep breath in through your right nostril for a count of four.

Gently press your right thumb against your right nostril.

Take a deep breath and hold it for a count of four.

Breathe out gently through your left nostril, counting to four as you do so.

Engage in this practice for 5-10 minutes, ensuring you keep a consistent pace.

Integrating these breathing exercises into your everyday life can enhance oxygen circulation to your cells, alleviate stress, and boost your overall wellness. For individuals with arthritis, effective breathing techniques can aid the body's inherent healing abilities, alleviate discomfort, and encourage a sense of calm.

CHAPTER 6

Lifestyle Changes

Consistent Movement: Advantages of Being Active

Engaging in consistent physical activity is vital for promoting overall health and wellness, especially for those dealing with arthritis. Participating in consistent physical activity can assist in alleviating arthritis symptoms, boosting joint function, and enriching overall well-being. Here are some important advantages of engaging in physical activity for those with arthritis:

1. Enhanced Joint Flexibility: Engaging in physical activity supports the maintenance and enhancement of joint flexibility, alleviating stiffness and expanding the range of motion. This holds great significance for those dealing with arthritis, as the stiffness in joints can greatly affect everyday tasks. Engaging in stretching exercises along with practices such as yoga and tai chi can greatly improve joint mobility.

2. Enhanced Muscular Support: Robust muscles offer improved support and stability to the joints, lowering the

likelihood of injury and easing discomfort in the joints. Engaging in resistance training and weight-bearing exercises is essential for developing and preserving muscle strength. Engaging in activities such as lifting weights, utilizing resistance bands, and performing bodyweight exercises can effectively enhance the strength of the muscles surrounding the impacted joints.

3. Weight Management: Keeping a healthy weight is essential for those with arthritis, as extra weight adds more pressure on weight-bearing joints such as the knees, hips, and spine. Engaging in consistent physical activity alongside a nutritious diet can support the attainment and upkeep of a healthy weight, easing the strain on the joints and providing relief from discomfort.

4. Reduced Inflammation: Engaging in physical activity can help lower inflammation levels by encouraging the release of substances that combat inflammation and boosting the body's inherent defenses against oxidative stress. This may assist in easing arthritis symptoms and enhancing overall well-being.

5. Boosted Mood and Mental Well-Being: Physical activity triggers the release of

endorphins, the body's own feel-good substances, which can alleviate discomfort and elevate spirits. Engaging in regular physical activity can help alleviate symptoms of depression and anxiety, often experienced by those living with arthritis. Participating in pleasurable pursuits such as walking, swimming, and dancing can greatly enhance one's mental well-being.

6. Boosted Vitality: Engaging in regular physical activity can effectively address tiredness, a frequent issue associated with arthritis. Engaging in physical activity enhances heart health and facilitates improved oxygen and nutrient flow to muscles and tissues, leading to a boost in overall energy levels.

7. Enhanced Rest: Engaging in physical activity can contribute to improved sleep quality by alleviating stress and encouraging a sense of calm. Improving sleep is crucial for alleviating arthritis symptoms and enhancing overall wellness.

When beginning a fitness journey, it's essential to select movements that are easy on the body and kind to the joints. Here are a few suggested activities for those dealing with arthritis:

Walking: An easy and beneficial method to maintain your activity levels. Walking promotes heart health, builds muscle strength, and increases flexibility in the joints.

Swimming: Engaging in water-based activities like swimming and water aerobics offers gentle resistance while being easy on the joints. The gentle embrace of the water cradles the body, minimizing the chance of harm.

Cycling: Engaging in either a stationary or traditional bicycle ride is a gentle yet effective way to enhance heart health and build strength in the lower body muscles.

Yoga and Tai Chi: These practices emphasize gentle stretching, balance, and a sense of calm. These options can promote better joint flexibility, alleviate stress, and boost overall wellness.

Before embarking on any exercise regimen, it's essential to seek guidance from a healthcare professional or physical therapist to confirm that the selected activities are safe and suitable for your individual circumstances. Methods for Easing Tension: Mindfulness Practices, Gentle Movement, and Relaxation Breathing

It's essential to handle stress effectively for those dealing with arthritis, as it can worsen symptoms and harm overall well-being. Integrating calming practices into your everyday life can enhance your mental and emotional health, lower inflammation, and ease the discomfort of arthritis. Here are some soothing methods to alleviate stress:

1. Meditation: This practice centers on honing your focus and clearing away distractions, leading to a serene state of relaxation and enhanced mental clarity. Consistent meditation practices can alleviate stress, anxiety, and depression, often experienced by those living with arthritis. Through fostering a sense of calm and awareness, meditation can assist in alleviating discomfort and enhancing overall health.

Ways to Engage in Mindfulness:

Seek out a serene and cozy spot where you can either sit or recline peacefully.

Gently close your eyes and inhale deeply, allowing your breaths to flow slowly and peacefully.

Concentrate on your breathing, a particular word or phrase, or a calming visual image.

Softly guide your attention back if your thoughts begin to drift.

Engage in this practice for 5-20 minutes each day, slowly extending the time as you grow more at ease.

2. Yoga: This practice harmonizes the body and mind through a blend of physical postures, breathing techniques, and meditation, fostering relaxation and enhancing overall well-being. Practicing yoga can enhance your joint flexibility, build muscle strength, and alleviate stress. This approach is especially advantageous for those dealing with arthritis, focusing on soft movements and conscious breathing.

Advantages of Practicing Yoga:

Enhances the ease of movement and expands the ability to bend and stretch.

Enhances muscle strength and promotes better balance.

Alleviates tension and encourages a sense of calm.

Boosts cognitive sharpness and promotes emotional health.

Varieties of Yoga:

Hatha Yoga: Emphasizes gentle movements and breathing practices, making it ideal for newcomers and those dealing with arthritis.

Restorative Yoga: Focuses on soothing relaxation and gentle stretching, utilizing props to provide support for the body in different poses.

Chair Yoga: Modifies classic yoga positions to be practiced while seated, ensuring accessibility for those with restricted movement.

3. Deep Breathing Techniques: Engaging in deep breathing techniques, often referred to as diaphragmatic breathing, can aid in alleviating stress, enhancing oxygen absorption, and fostering a sense of calm. These exercises are easy to incorporate into your routine and can be performed in any setting.

Ways to Engage in Deep Breathing:

Find a cozy spot to either sit or recline comfortably.

Gently rest one hand on your chest and the other on your belly.

Take a deep breath in through your nose, letting your belly expand as you fill your lungs with fresh air. Keep your chest as calm and steady as possible.

Breathe out gently through your mouth, letting your belly relax as you let the air go.

Engage in this practice for 5-10 minutes, concentrating on slow, calming breaths.

Integrating these calming practices into your everyday life can assist in alleviating arthritis symptoms, boost mental and emotional health, and elevate your overall quality of life.
The Significance of Sleep and Relaxation

Rest and sleep play a vital role in handling arthritis and supporting overall well-being. Getting enough sleep and rest helps the body heal and rejuvenate, minimizing inflammation and easing discomfort. For those dealing with arthritis, emphasizing sleep and rest is essential for alleviating symptoms and enhancing overall well-being.

1. Rest: Restful slumber is essential for holistic health and wellness. It supports the body's ability to heal tissues, balance hormones, and sustain mental clarity. Inadequate sleep can worsen arthritis symptoms, heighten pain sensitivity, and adversely affect mood and energy levels.

Suggestions for Enhancing Rest:

Set a Regular Sleep Routine: Aim to go to bed and rise at the same time each day, including weekends, to help harmonize your body's natural rhythms.

Establish a Soothing Nighttime Ritual: Participate in tranquil activities prior to sleep, like enjoying a good book, soaking in a warm bath, or employing relaxation methods.

Establish a Restful Atmosphere: Make sure your sleeping space is comfortably cool, dimly lit, and peaceful. Opt for a cozy mattress and pillows that provide gentle support for your joints.

Reduce Caffeine and Alcohol Intake: Steer clear of caffeine and alcohol in the hours leading up to bedtime, as they may disrupt your sleep quality.

Minimize Screen Exposure: Cut back on the use of screens (like phones, tablets, and TVs) in the evening, since the blue light they emit can interfere with your natural sleep patterns.

2. Rest: Alongside quality sleep, taking breaks during the day is crucial for alleviating arthritis symptoms and avoiding fatigue. Taking time to rest

helps the body heal and minimizes the chances of flare-ups and heightened discomfort.

Suggestions for Embracing Relaxation:

Pay Attention to Your Body: Listen to your body's cues and allow yourself to rest when necessary to prevent fatigue.

Take it easy: Divide your tasks into smaller, more manageable parts and switch between doing something and taking a break to avoid feeling worn out.

Engage in Soft Stretching: Integrate soft stretching movements into your daily routine to ease tension and minimize stiffness.

Incorporate supportive tools: Embrace the use of supportive tools like braces, canes, or ergonomic implements to ease the strain on your joints and help you save energy.

By emphasizing the importance of sleep and rest, those dealing with arthritis can better handle their symptoms, lessen pain and inflammation, and enhance their overall quality of life. Integrating consistent physical activity, methods to alleviate stress, and ensuring adequate sleep and relaxation into your daily routine can contribute to joint wellness, boost both physical and mental health, and encourage a more vibrant, active lifestyle.

THE END

Printed in Dunstable, United Kingdom

73869753R00036